Vignettes of Yvette at Vi

A Love Story of a Husband for His Wife

John G. Gurley

AuthorHouse™
1663 Liberty Drive
Bloomington, IN 47403
www.authorhouse.com
Phone: 1 (800) 839-8640

Published by AuthorHouse 01/26/2015

ISBN: 978-1-4969-6504-2 (sc)
ISBN: 978-1-4969-6528-8 (e)

Library of Congress Control Number: 2015901189

INTRODUCTION

On Carmen's day off each week, Marcela Montalvo takes excellent care of Yvette. After Marcela read most of these Vignettes, she told me: "It is a love story." Oh, that is so right! I offer you these Vignettes as a reflection of my love for Yvette as she was and for Yvette as she presently is. It really is simple: it's a love story.

VIGNETTES OF YVETTE AT Vi

1

Two weeks after our 67th wedding anniversary, on a morning in early April, 2012, two nurses came to our apartment and took my wife, Yvette, away. For the past four or five years, Yvette had been steadily slipping away from me, on her own, as she was being drawn into the tentacles of dementia. I knew that the two nurses were coming, of course, for I had arranged it.

But, when they led her out of the door of our apartment, and Yvette turned her head to look back at me, with a puzzled and then a frightened look, I told her that everything would be fine, blew her a kiss, closed the door — and then I cried my heart out. I collapsed — yes, a 92-year-old weakling collapsed, but a weakling still head over heels in love. Then, I told myself to think of Yvette, not me. What must she be going through now, being led away from her home by two strangers, to God knows where? Those thoughts did not quiet me down. Afterwards, I kept seeing that frightened look, as Yvette struggled to turn back to me, for many, many weeks, day and night.

2

The two nurses did not have to take Yvette very far. Her Memory Support unit was in the Care Center, a large, two-story building next door to our retirement home, now called by the funny name of Vi at Palo Alto. We are in the northwest corner of the sprawling campus of Stanford University. If you stand facing Vi's Care Center, the entry door on the left says Skilled Nursing. The one on the right says Assisted Living. There is no indication anywhere of the two Memory Support (MS) units. Dementia is apparently a dirty word. It is also a coded word, for to reach MS

1, you go through the Assisted Living door, turn right to a coded door that will open only if you punch the correct five keys, in the right order. To get to MS 2, you walk through all of MS 1 to a second coded door that puts you into an area with utility rooms and public toilets. Finally, there is a third coded door that lets you into MS 2. So MS 2 is really hidden away. That is where the two nurses were taking my wife. That is where Yvette is presumably to remain for the rest of her life.

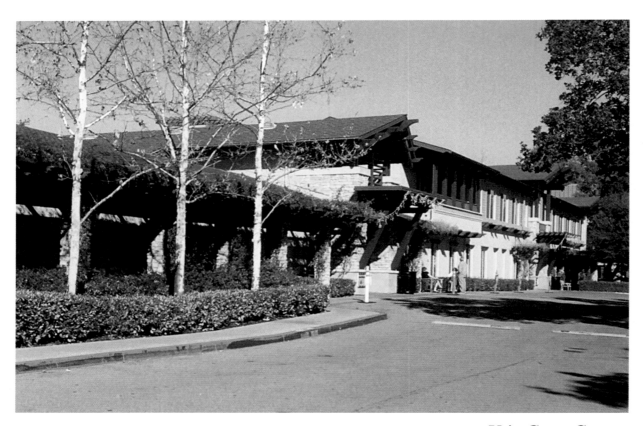

Vi's Care Center

3

Each Memory Support unit has an inner, walled-in garden with a cement path meandering through and around it. For the first three or four months this is where Yvette wanted to be. So several times each day, I put my hand on her upper arm and guided her 'round and 'round the garden. We walked for five minutes or so, then sat on a bench for less than a minute, up again, and so on. Yvette was there because she thought that once she got outside she could find a way to escape her confinement.

There were two locked gates in our garden, one leading to the inner garden of the other Memory Support unit, and the other leading into a much larger garden for those in Assisted Living. Yvette had found these two partly-hidden gates the first day she was there. Each round of our garden walks included a stop at these gates — to see if they were still locked, as they had been a minute or two earlier. Twice on different days during these early months. Yvette found the gate unlocked that ushered us into the inner garden of the other Memory Support unit. Though she seemed greatly encouraged by this, it was actually a dead end, for there were no other gates in this garden, and the only door led into MS 1 itself, where the residents were just as confined as Yvette was. But we kept at it, day after day, several times a day, for months. When it came time for me to leave at the end of each day, Yvette, using her last hope, would say to me plaintively: "Please, please take me with you. Please." How would you feel if you were confronted with that? That's how I felt.

4

As we walked in the garden, I held Yvette's upper arm, or sometimes simply her hand, for a good reason. She had taken several bad falls during the previous eight years. The first was on a morning walk with her friends. The next while playing tennis. Two others were on morning walks after we moved into the retirement home from our campus house. Another was on a San Francisco sidewalk when we were going to a restaurant. The last was coming out of a museum in San Francisco, and that entailed a 911 call and 10 hours in a San Francisco hospital. Every fall of Yvette's was on cement, on her face or head, for she was apparently unable to break these falls with her hands and arms. No concussions, however, were revealed from these spills.

That's why I had to be careful on our garden walks. I became convinced, despite the several negative brain scans, that Yvette's growing dementia had to be related to these frequent crashes on her face and head. Then, as time went on, Yvette was finding it increasingly difficult to sit down and to rise from a seated position. She was also walking less confidently, with more hesitation. Finally, she wasn't able to walk at all. She was confined to a transport chair.

I admit how slow I was in realizing that I had the whole thing backwards. Yvette's dementia was the cause of her falls. The falls did not cause the dementia. Dementia is not entirely mental deterioration. It is equally physical, too. Yvette's brain was no longer giving her adequate instructions on how to walk. Then her brain shut down instructions on how to hold and handle utensils while eating. Her speech was less distinct. Even swallowing food properly requires clear commands from the brain. During the past year, I would say that Yvette has held her own mentally, but physically she has gone downhill. No-one would claim that dementia is entirely a physical ailment, but you had better keep your eyes open for all sorts of physical disabilities if a loved one develops dementia.

5

When Yvette and I moved into this retirement home, then called Classic Residence by Hyatt and now renamed Vi at Palo Alto, in the Fall of 2005, a man named Fitz Corey lived in an apartment close by. Early on, Fitz invited us in to see some of his unusual pieces of furniture, and over the next year or so we frequently saw him in the Bistro having breakfast. Yvette and I thought that he was a very pleasant neighbor. Yvette never missed a chance to talk to him.

Then one morning, after Fitz had had some sort of illness, Yvette and I saw him sitting outdoors on a bench, presumably waiting for a valet to bring up his car. The only trouble was that all he had on was a hat and his undershorts. Not even shoes or socks. We and, I would guess, plenty of others, reported this to our front desk. Within a few days, Fitz was transferred from his apartment to one in Assisted Living, located on the second floor of the Care Center.

Soon, a PDA (Private Duty Aide) was hired by Fitz's family to care for him several hours each day. This PDA was Carmen Galindo, who had been born in Buenos Aires, had come to this country as a university graduate student, and now lived with her mother and a brother in Redwood City. Carmen cared for Fitz for several years, until he died in 2012. Carmen thus became free at precisely the time I decided that I could no longer tend to Yvette ten hours a day and needed help. So Yvette's friend Fitz — or his family— found Carmen, then died and released Carmen to Yvette, just when Yvette's own dementia required it. That's how Carmen eventually became, in my imagination, my adopted granddaughter.

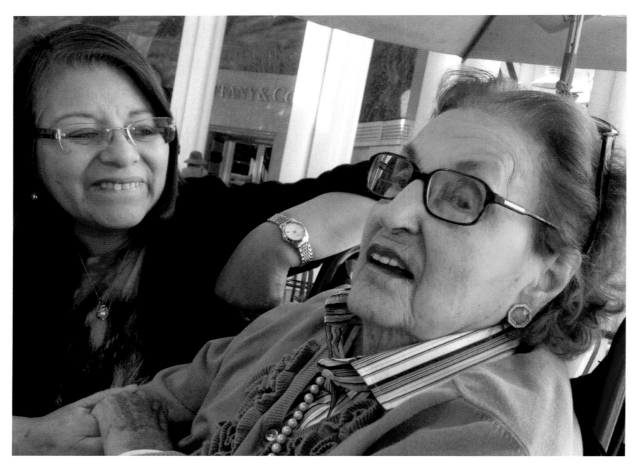

Carmen and Yvette

6

Many of Yvette's friends began to leave her as she sunk lower into dementia's quicksand. This is meant in two senses. Yvette began to forget some of her friends — and so they departed from her memory. But these were few at first compared to those friends who simply chose not to see her anymore. "I wish to remember her as she was." "I didn't think they let non-family into the Care Center." Mostly though, departure was accompanied by silence. Several friends just disappeared without a sound. However, that says nothing special about Yvette. It seems to be just par for the course. The Memory Support units have many largely abandoned people.

Nevertheless, at the time, I was disappointed that virtually none of Yvette's friends came in to see her. As time went on, these departed friends meant less and less, for Yvette was carrying out the departures in her own mind: she was forgetting her friends. If some of her friends had come over to see her, Yvette surely would have remembered them longer. When they silently departed, Yvette had only me to speak their names and remind her of her pals. I did my best but there was no way that I could substitute for actual companions. Memory Support requires support from friends and family, but, while that is by no means absent, it is unusual enough for an observer to feel pity for all those who are neglected and left to die without the warmth of friends and family.

7

Even at the age of 91, Yvette is a very pretty lady. Carmen, each morning, with her skill and passion, enhances Yvette's beauty by dressing her in lovely, matching clothes, all newly washed and ironed by Carmen herself. Once each week, Carmen takes Yvette to the beauty salon that is in the Care Center for whatever is necessary to keep Yvette's hair looking good. Yes, Carmen works hard at it, but she has a 91-year-old beauty queen underneath it all.

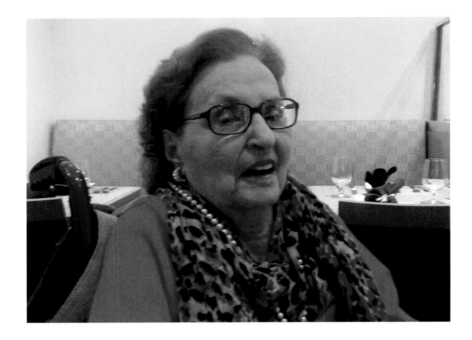

When Carmen, Yvette (in her transport chair), and I stroll through the Care Center, as we do for half an hour or so each day, several employees along the way invariably stop what they're doing and come over to say hello to Yvette and tell her how very pretty she looks. Carmen and I believe that Yvette enjoys the attention. Yvette usually has a big smile for these admirers. And, let me tell you — from, of course, an impartial observer — that when Yvette smiles, the whole world swoons. Yvette has a nightgown that says on the front of it: The Queen of Absolutely Everything. I got this for her because I know the truth when I see it. I hope you will excuse the hubris.

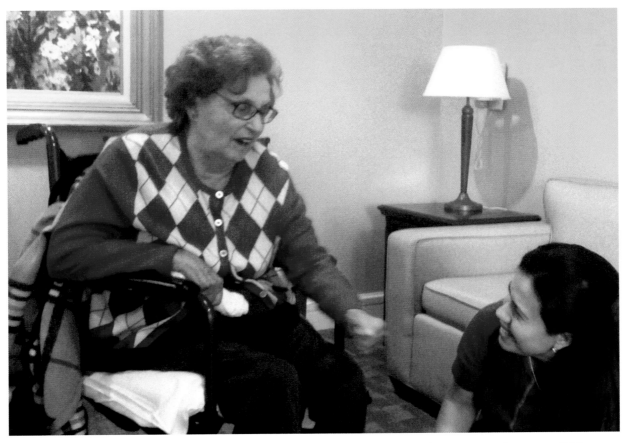

Marcela Montalvo and Yvette

8

Yvette recently contracted aspiration pneumonia in both lungs, caused by mis-swallowing food that ended up lodged in her lungs. At that time, Yvette's doctor was on vacation, so another doctor came over, with x-ray results in hand. After prescribing antibiotics for Yvette, and discussing her situation with the nurse, he turned to me and said that we should do everything to make Yvette comfortable, for that's about all we can do under these circumstances. Then he left abruptly.

That suggested to me that Yvette was going to die, and the best we could do was to make her dying comfortable. Carmen and I did not buy that, but, what is much more important, neither did Yvette. She refused to die, fighting her way through the pneumonia to a successful conclusion. Yvette seemed stronger to us after she beat the pneumonia than she had been prior to the disease.

That doctor's "comfortable advice" was still bugging me when our own Dr. Henry Jones returned to his office. I had to talk to him about something pertaining to Yvette. During our telephone conversation, I was dismayed to hear him say, not once but four or five times, that from here on out what we want to do is to make Yvette as comfortable as possible. I mentioned what really good shape she was in, and his response was to be thankful for that while it lasts — the implication being that this could be a very brief period.

The next day, I sent Dr. Jones an e-mail expressing how upset I was at the end of our telephone conversation. I told him that Carmen and I — I should have added the nursing staff, too — worked very hard every single day, not just for the comfort of Yvette, but to improve her both mentally and physically. We take her almost every day to the Stanford Shopping Center, where we discuss the shoppers and their bags, the small kids running by, the dogs sniffing their way along. I try to relate anything we see to some past event in Yvette's life. During the hours in the Care Center, we run videos of musical programs, both pop and classical, often operatic duets or ensembles. I discuss with Yvette where we were when we heard Pavarotti sing in a certain opera. And so on, every day. I told him how Carmen flexes Yvette's legs in bicycle fashion before getting her up each morning. How Carmen has encouraged Yvette to use her legs to move herself while in her chair. Every day Carmen gets another staff member to help her stand Yvette up on her feet and then walk with Yvette as far as Yvette is able to go. Then a short rest, and do it again. And again. Carmen and I think that Yvette is improving both mentally and physically from our efforts.

Dr. Jones readily agreed that Carmen's and my efforts, with the nursing staff's contributions added in, have been the most important thing in Yvette's present life. Okay, I probably misunderstood our doctor in our telephone talk. If so, my apologies. What is clear, however, is that Carmen's and my own health depend partly — largely?— on our belief that we are helping Yvette, for all our days are spent to achieve that objective. Anything like comfort talk threatens what we feel we are achieving — better health for Yvette. It also threatens our own health. That's why we explode when we think we have heard more comfort talk.

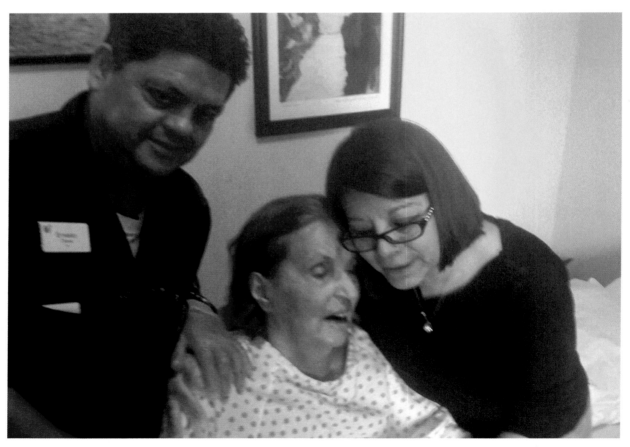

Ernesto Chavez and Carmen after Yvette's pneumonia.

9

From about 1970 to 2010, Yvette and I had season tickets each year to the San Francisco Opera and to the San Francisco Symphony performances. That's the music that Yvette still has in her ear. In a sense, that music is in her eyes, too. At the Opera, we had front row seats for two reasons: to see the musicians as they played, and to see more clearly — without using binoculars — the opera singers. At the Symphony, our seats were on the side terrace, which gave us a wonderful view of virtually all the musicians, and of the conductor, as well.

For Yvette, therefore, we need more than a radio; we require videos of classical and operatic performances. There are several ways to get these, but Carmen and I each have an iPad, and that is what we prop up before Yvette when we believe she will enjoy hearing and watching musical performances. Sometimes this is at meal times, which means that Carmen and Yvette cannot take their places at their dining table — which would impose their music on others — but must eat in Yvette's room. Since Yvette's bout with aspiration pneumonia, her food has been liquid or puréed. So all of Yvette's food comes in small containers, requiring no cutting or other preparation, and this makes it easier for Carmen to feed Yvette in what would otherwise be cramped quarters. Yvette watches and listens, sitting upright, and opening her mouth from time to time for the puréed food. Pretty soft!

One sacrifice that this practice entails is that Yvette forgoes the pleasure of eating next to Donna Sommer, a former pediatrician at Kaiser Permanente, and who loves Yvette. She gives Yvette presents occasionally, inquires of Carmen how Yvette is doing, and comments to me and others about Yvette's nice appearance that day.

Yvette's seat is at one end of a table that accommodates six diners. Donna, or the doctor as she is often called, sits next to Yvette's end on Yvette's left. Carmen feeds Yvette from Yvette's right. This set-up enables Donna to watch Yvette, as she often does, to speak to her in her very soft voice, and even, once in a while, to hold hands with her. Donna believes that Yvette is the daughter of Carmen, even though there is a half century between them going the other way. Yvette and Donna communicate with each other with their eyes, through Carmen's very liberal translation of what each has said to the other, and by holding hands. They have plenty of time for all that during the meal, for Donna eats practically nothing while Yvette has only to open her mouth for the food intakes, leaving her hands free.

So Yvette has two interesting places for eating her meals. One in her room with Carmen and the music that continues to capture her attention, and the other in the dining room, where Donna attempts to communicate in an almost inaudible voice. If Yvette responds, her message is often inarticulate. This requires a translator, and here is where Carmen shines. Carmen explains to one of them that the other just said that she loves you. Later, the same translation goes the other way. Carmen knows what they're saying, and it is always "I love you."

That's the translator that everyone needs.

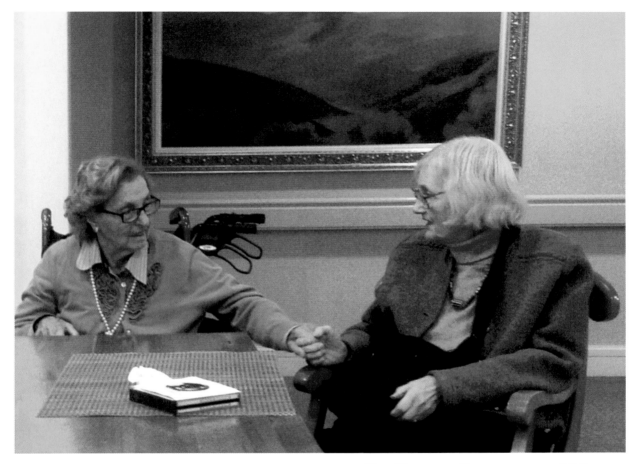

Dr. Donna Sommer and Yvette

10

Dementia embraces both mental and physical disabilities. After all, the brain is involved in both areas. Yvette, very early on, began having difficulties with writing. It wasn't long before she could no longer write her own name properly, in cursive style. I encouraged her to print, but this helped for only a short time, and then even that was soon gone. It took a few more years before her speaking became less and less articulate. Now, much of what she says Carmen and I cannot understand. For a long while, this apparently caused Yvette to speak less and less. We had months of almost total silence from Yvette, though she learned to speak with her eyes, with facial expressions, and with vocal tones suggesting agitation, pleasure, annoyance, and so on.

Carmen and I began a campaign to reverse these trends, by asking questions of Yvette, encouraging her to answer, or by making some statement that might compel her to respond. We kept at it, for weeks and months, and sure enough Yvette began to open up. She started responding to what we said, and we pretended to understand everything she said. "Oh, yes?," we said. "Yes," she would answer. Then something quite clear would greet us. Her articulation began to improve. During the past several months, Yvette has been talking more, and perhaps a fourth of it we can understand.

So when we hear something clear and loud from Yvette, we take note. A few days ago, when she first saw me in the afternoon, she said to Carmen: "Do you know him? He's a professor." A week before that, as Yvette was exercising in the family room by back-pedaling in her chair, she said to me, as she was moving away, "I'll be back again." Today, as we entered the family room, I said to Carmen and Yvette: "Here we are in the gym for Yvette's exercise program." Yvette immediately responded, looking at Carmen, "Now we're both happy." The meaning was a little fuzzy, but it was said clearly. She has pronounced the names of several people very clearly, who stop to talk to her, by reading their badges. "Francesca" was a bit difficult, but Yvette got it. When people crowded ahead of us at a traffic light crossing, Yvette yelled at them "What about us?" Several times, while we were seated at La

Baguette watching the passing parade, Yvette has suddenly said, while pointing, "Look at that!"

For those of you now yawning at these examples, I must tell you that Carmen and I are thrilled to hear Yvette talk again. Each time we hear something that is wonderful and clear, at least one of us gives Yvette a great big hug. It simply doesn't always have to be downhill all the way.

11

I am not sure where Yvette got all her present strength. She did play tennis most of her life, very good tennis. She was a lefty, with a fine forehand, and, on her right side, a two-handed backhand. That may explain the super-strength she now has with her left arm. Despite not walking for over a year now, Yvette still retains lots of strength in her legs. This is partly owing to Carmen's daily efforts to that end. But Yvette also did an hour of body exercises each day for forty years, using weights on her ankles and wrists. That must still count for something. Anyway, there are many members of the nursing staff in Memory Support who have encountered Yvette's strength, especially in her left arm, and have commented on it.

Yvette is not always smiling. She can get a determined look in her eyes and in the way she sets her mouth, presumably in preparation for a slugfest with whoever happens to be tormenting her at the moment. These days her hands are in fist positions, so all she has to do when she sees a fight brewing is raise her left arm, with fist in place, threatening a left upper-cut to her opponent's chin or a left hook into the body. This is the usual scene when Yvette is awakened from a nap and is being moved from the bed to her chair. Then, for a minute or two, it is, for Yvette, all-out warfare on those enemy forces daring to disturb her.

Over a year ago, when Yvette was on a tranquilizer, she reacted to it by being more combative than ever, and these aggressive moods lasted longer, over hours. Once she was taken off this medication, while her combativeness persisted, she could now be talked out of it in minutes. Instead of a threatening left hook, a little talk quickly turns that into a more friendly gesture — a rubbing of her hand on the cheek of her ex-tormentor, or a relaxed arm ready for hand-holding. Still, the staff has to be careful of the awesome strength that Yvette still retains in her arms and legs.

During the last year or so when Yvette and I were living together in our apartment, I encountered her strength many times. She became reluctant to taking showers, and so I had to use not only my best persuasion but, at times, a bit of force to get her into the shower. A few times she reacted to this by suddenly swinging me around until I landed on the floor, much as a wrestler would who wanted to pin his opponent's shoulders to the mat. In this period, Yvette was continually trying to escape from our apartment, not for any specific destination but simply to get out. I had to get an alarm put inside our door to warn me when Yvette had opened the door for an escape. Then, perhaps from the bathroom, I had to rush down the corridor, and sometimes down a couple of corridors, to catch up to her. Then I had the problem of persuasion versus force to get her back, and here again I came face to face with her tremendous strength.

This problem is now so much easier to deal with. We all still have to be on our toes to avoid a left upper-cut to the chin from an angry woman, but we also know how easy it is to turn that threatening blow into a gesture of love. Carmen has told me about a whack on the head followed immediately by a kiss. We all hope

that before long there will prevail only the kiss.

12

Does Yvette still know me as her husband, or as some guy who has been around here a lot recently? That question is with me almost every day. I'm thinking: Of course, in a way, Yvette knows me. I've been here almost every day for 22 months. But does she know that she's married to me? Not to mention the 68 years. When she sees me, she usually smiles. I love those smiles, but I don't count them as definitive, since she smiles at many people. I may simply be a familiar face.

However, I do think she still knows who I really am. Every once in a while, Yvette will look straight at me and say: "Hi, dearie." That's a greeting she has used for several decades when seeing me. She said that as recently as a week ago. I have been using this form of greeting, too, to her, hoping to see her react knowingly to it. She has, with a big smile, though not all of the time. But when Yvette says "Hi, dearie," even if only once in a month, I know for sure that she knows me as her husband.

I have also told her a hundred times — I'm not kidding— about how we met at the Sutter Lawn Tennis Club in Sacramento and that we were married at my parents' home in Sacramento. This almost always brings forth a beautiful smile, one that I interpret as a smile of remembrance. However, is she remembering the actual events or remembering that I've told her the same story before? It's a pretty good bet it's the former. But "Hi, dearie," is a better bet.

Yvette also refers to me as "Jack" occasionally, which she has used for almost 70 years. She will ask Carmen, when I have lagged behind on one of our daily walks, "Is Jack coming?" Carmen mentions my name to Yvette several times every day. "Jack will be here in a few minutes." When Carmen and Yvette are in the bathroom, and I have just arrived and am sitting on the sofa in her room, I have heard Carmen say many times "Jack is here. We're all going to Stanford [Shopping Center]." So Yvette does know me as Jack, and I count that as a big plus — for she does not mention anyone else by name, even Carmen.

Vignettes of Yvette at Vi

Yvette seems to have a good memory of my sister, Helen, who lives far away in the Dominican Republic. Since Yvette has been in Memory Support, she has seen Helen only twice, each time off and on over a week. Her memory of Helen seems to go back quite a way. This works in my favor, for I am of course associated with Helen and am the one frequently telling Yvette the latest stories about Helen, which Yvette always seems interested in. When Yvette is fidgeting and making vocal sounds to accompany the fidgeting, I can always stop her by telling her something about Helen. Hardly anything else works. If Yvette has Helen in mind, she certainly has me in mind, too.

I don't know how many times I have told Yvette our entire history together, all in five minutes or less each time. Marriage in Sacramento, graduate studies at Stanford, teaching and research at

Princeton, doing research in Washington, D. C., and then back to Stanford. I have reminded her frequently of what she accomplished before meeting me: graduated from San Diego State; completed an IBM course, in Ithaca, New York, on computers; sent to Sacramento to maintain the State's array of huge computers, lodged in two spacious rooms. These frequent discussions are mainly meant to remind her of herself, and to try to keep fresh in her memory the main events in her life. So much the better if they also remind her that I'm her husband.

13

I believe that the very last thing that Yvette did on her own, before sinking a bit too far into her dementia, was to take her credit card and walk over to Nordstrom's to purchase two pairs of pajamas for me. When she returned with her purchases, I remember that I was surprised to hear her explain, in so much detail, how she decided on a winter and a summer purchase of PJs, how she signed the credit card receipt, the walk over there and back, and other particulars of the outing. However, later, when her dementia was there for all to see, including me, I wondered if she had had some premonition of the difficulties to come when she so proudly told me of her accomplishments at Nordstrom's. Yvette may have been a few steps ahead of me.

In any case, I wear one or the other of the PJs every night to bed. And that's when I tell Yvette — yes, out loud — what a very fine job she did in purchasing them all by herself. Every night I think that she should know that.

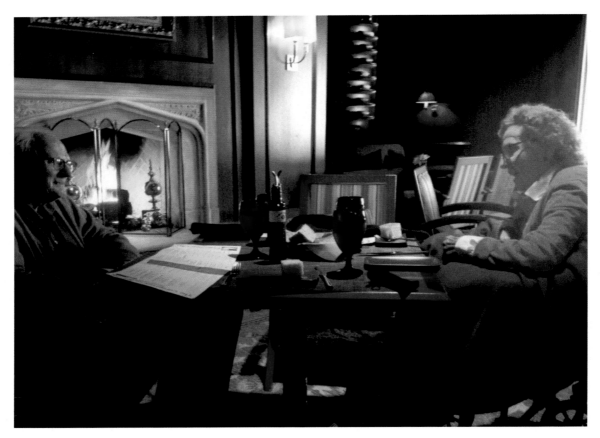

Jack and Yvette, Half Moon Bay, June, 2013

Printed in the United States
By Bookmasters